Dr. Walsh's Simple Solutions To Back Pain!

*New Smyrna Beach Chiropractor
Dr. Donald B. Walsh III Reveals
Simple Solutions To Treat and
Prevent Back Pain*

Dr. Donald B. Walsh III

First Printing, 2010

ISBN 978-1456308605

Printed in the United States of America

DISCLAIMER

About the author

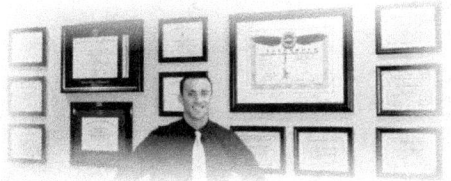

Dr. Donald B. Walsh III owns and operates the New Smyrna Spine & Injury Center in Florida. He is an Honors graduate of Palmer College of Chiropractic, Florida and The University of North Florida. He also earned both a Diplomate and a Fellowship in Acupuncture from the International Academy of Medical Acupuncture.

Dr. Walsh holds certification in Auto Accident Injury Trauma, Mild Traumatic Brain Injury, Auto Safety, and in the Cox® Flexion/Distraction technique.

Dr. Walsh is credentialed through the Florida Bar to provide continuing education credits for attorneys and their paralegal staff.

Dr. Walsh leads a physically active lifestyle and practices what he preaches. When he is not busy with patients or advancing his education, you will often find him with his 4 year old son exercising in the gym, surfing in the ocean, playing semi-pro baseball or training in Jiu-Jitsu.

Table of Contents

The Basics

What Is Back Pain?

Back pain (also called dorsalgia) is pain felt in the back that usually originates from the muscles, nerves, bones, tendons, ligaments, joints or other structures of and in the spine.

Symptoms of back pain may include:

- Muscle ache

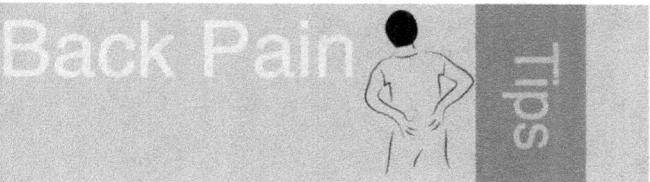

- Shooting or stabbing pain
- Pain that radiates down your leg
- Limited flexibility or range of motion of your back
- Inability to stand straight

Back pain is one of the two most common reasons for visiting a doctor. It is second only to the common cold.

Who Gets Back Pain?

It is estimated that over 90% of Americans will experience one or more episodes of back pain in their lifetime.

Men and women, young and old, and every nationality can experience low back pain.

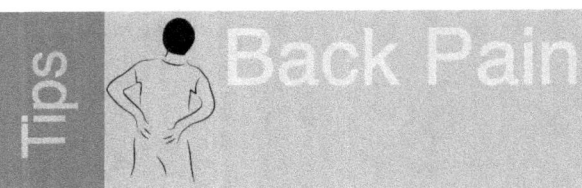

Certain occupations are more prone to back pain than others. People who sit or stand in one position for long periods of time, people who constantly bend over or reach up and/or down while in awkward positions, and people who have high stress jobs all have higher instances of back pain.

A Common Cause Of Doctor Visits

Back pain accounts for almost half of all doctor visits in the United States.

It is also one of the leading causes of missed work, second only to the common cold and flu.

According to the latest study in the

Back Pain Tips

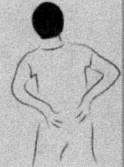

Journal of the American Medical Association (JAMA Feb13, 2008) the cost to American's exceeded $85 billion in 2005 alone. This amount does not include the cost of lost productivity that industry experienced from absences related to back pain.

What Causes Back Pain In People?

The number one most common cause of back pain is lumbar muscle strain.

Patients may or may not remember the initial event that triggered their muscle spasm, but the good news is that with proper care, most episodes

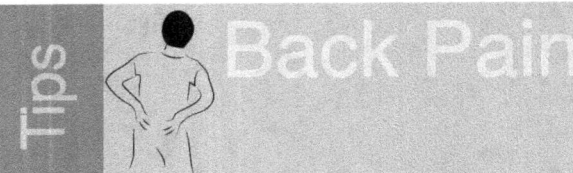

of back pain from muscle strains will resolve completely within a few weeks.

The Second Most Common Cause Of Back Pain Is...

The number two most common cause of back pain is a ruptured disc. A ruptured disc is also called a herniated disc.

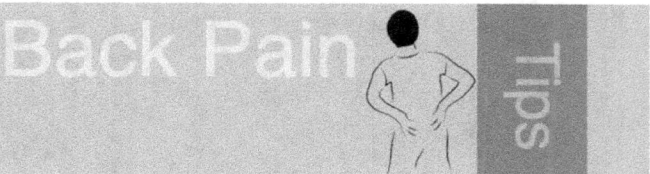

How to treat the back pain from a herniated disc depends on the particular individual and situation. However, it always requires the care of a doctor well educated and experienced in spinal care.

Typically this would be a chiropractor for conservative care and a neurosurgeon for surgical care.

Back Pain Can Be Caused By Spinal Stenosis

Spinal stenosis is a condition in which the spinal canal narrows and compresses the spinal cord and nerves.

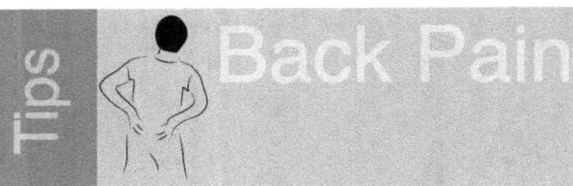

Spinal stenosis is usually a result of spinal degeneration (arthritis) that occurs as we grow older.

But, it could also be caused by osteoporosis, a tumor, a disc bulge, disc herniation, infection, dislocation, fracture, scoliosis, spondylolisthesis, ligamentum flavum hypertrophy or inflammation from a traumatic event.

Sciatica Is Another Common Complaint With Back Pain

Many people call back pain sciatica but this is not always an accurate description

Sciatica is pressure on the actual

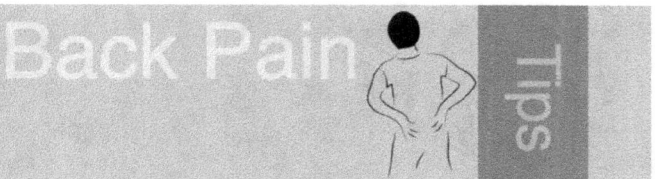

sciatic nerve which runs from your low back all the way down your leg to the tips of your toes. Sciatica is usually caused by disk herniations and/or spinal stenosis.

People who experience sciatica often have back pain as well as pain or numbness that travels down the back of the leg and into the ankle and foot.

Your Pelvis Can Be Causing Your Low Back Pain

At the base of your spine is your pelvis and this part of the body has many muscles and nerves going to and from the area.

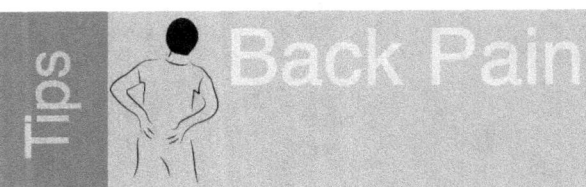

A misalignment of your pelvis can cause back pain and even pain that radiates or travels down your leg thereby mimicking sciatica.

Is It Really Old Age?

We are told that as we age we should expect more pain because arthritis is part of the aging process.

This is not necessarily true. Many people do develop arthritis as they age but this is not the result of the aging process. It is the result of the cumulative effect of the hundreds or

Back Pain Tips

thousands of micro traumas to our spines that we have experienced.

Fortunately, arthritis is preventable and, even if you do have arthritis, it is usually treatable.

Bulging Discs

Bulging discs in the spine are a form of arthritis. They are caused by an injury to one or more of the spinal discs that was never treated or fixed.

Because of the lack of treatment, over time the discs lose water and nutrients which causes them to become both flatter and wider.

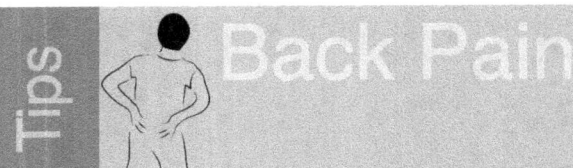

This can cause the disc to put pressure directly on the nerves or cause irritation to other tissues which causes the body to produce chemicals that can cause pain.

Such A Small Muscle For Such A Big Pain

The periformis muscle, which attaches from your tailbone to your hip, can be a major source of back pain.

In fact, if you have a severe enough case you may even show the clinical

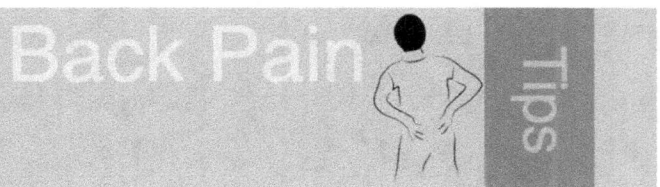

signs and symptoms of a disc herniation with pain and numbness radiating down the leg.

This is called pseudo-sciatica.

Don't Slip!

Slipping on a smooth surface and landing on your backside can be a major pain in the rear. If not properly cared for, these types of injuries can produce severe and long term pain.

While it may be just a bruise, it could also be a herniated disc, or worse, a fracture of your spine.

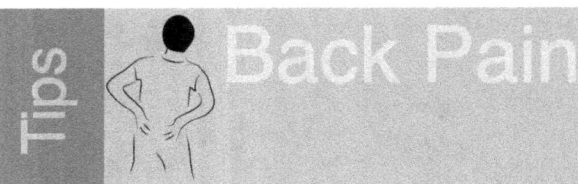

So watch where you walk and be careful on slippery surfaces. If you do fall and experience pain, have it checked by a spine expert.

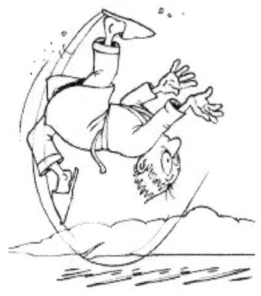

Car Accidents

Car and motorcycle accidents are another very common cause of back and neck pain which affects millions of people every year.

Consider that a motor vehicle is a big chunk of metal weighing about 5,000 pounds and travelling 5 or 10 miles per hour, maybe even faster. A motor

Back Pain Tips

vehicle is stronger and has less flexibility than a human body. That's why, when a human is struck by a vehicle, the body is bent, bruised and broken and the vehicle sustains minimal damage.

Your pain is due to the blunt and the piercing traumas these incredible wrenching forces create in, and cause to, your body.

Basic Anatomy

The spine is made up of bones, ligaments, discs, tendons, muscles, and nerves. Each one plays a specific role and each one can be the cause of your back pain.

Your spine is what holds you upright. It protects your spinal cord.

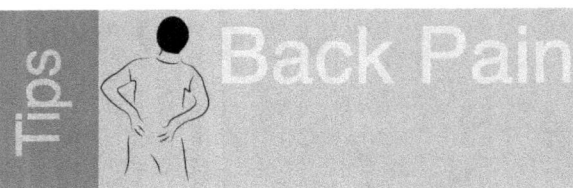

It is what allows you to move and be flexible.

It is a truly remarkable piece of engineering.

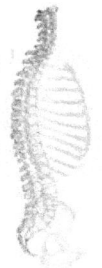

Bones

Your spine is made up of 24 movable bones called vertebra and 5 fused bones called the sacrum.

These bones are what support our weight, allow us to be flexible, and protect our spine.

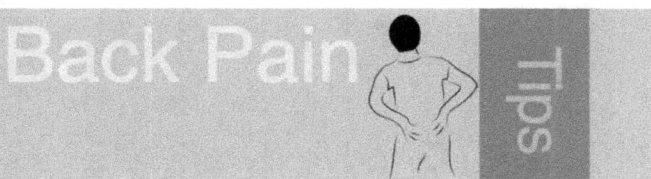

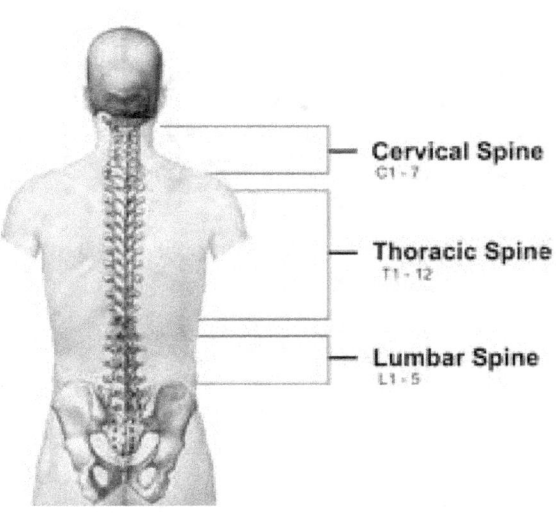

Cervical Spine
C1 - 7

Thoracic Spine
T1 - 12

Lumbar Spine
L1 - 5

Ligaments

Ligaments are the strong connective tissue that holds our bones together and in place. They are stronger than steel of the same thickness.

They have very little stretching ability and can take a long time to heal when injured.

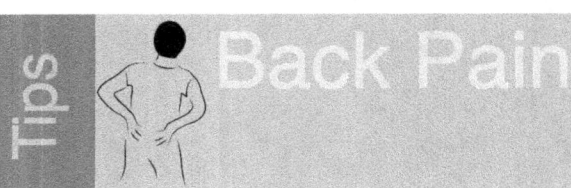

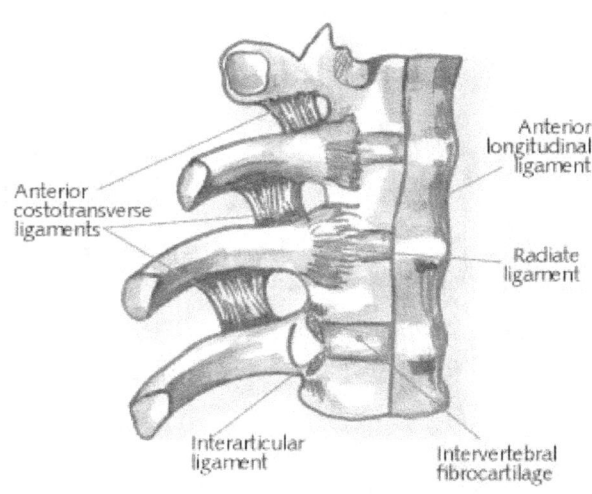

Anterior longitudinal ligament

Anterior costotransverse ligaments

Radiate ligament

Interarticular ligament

Intervertebral fibrocartilage

The Magical Miraculous Disc

The intervertebral disc is a very crucial part of the spine. It is often the part that is causing the symptoms and can be debilitating at times.

The disc is comprised of two

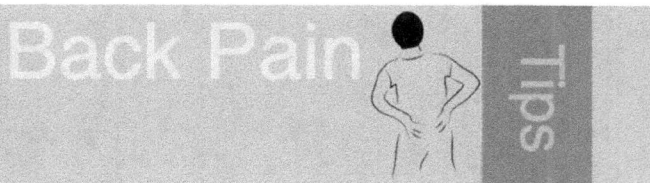

components.

The outer most part is called the annulus fibrosus and is made up of overlapping layers of connective tissue. The connective tissue that makes up the annulus fibrosis is a very strong yet flexible material.

The inner most part is called the nucleus pulposus. The material is a

viscous jelly like substance that is
used as a shock absorber.

When you herniate a disc, the
nucleus pulposus pushes the
annulus fibrosus in a direction that it
should not go.

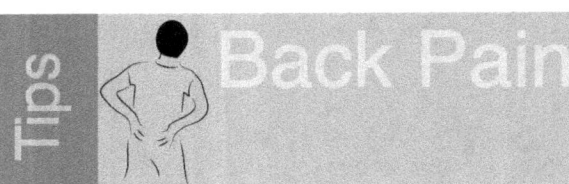

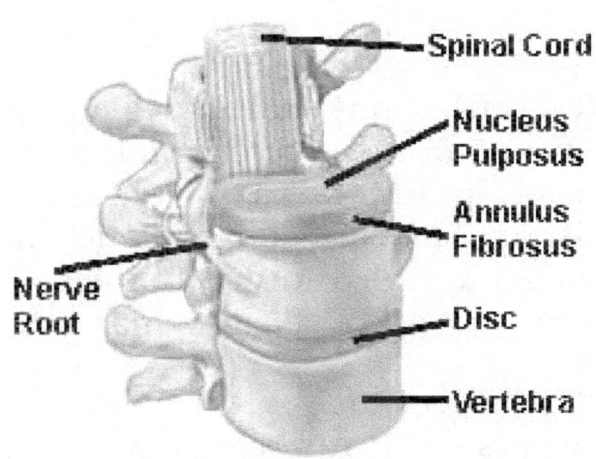

Muscles And Tendons

You cannot talk about muscles without talking about tendons and vice versa.

The muscles are what allow us to move around. They are the power to do things.

The tendons are what attach the

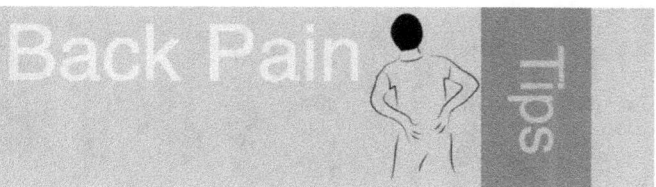

muscles to the bones.

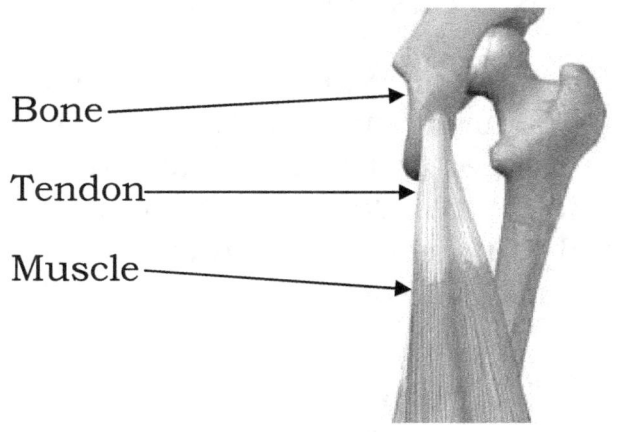

Bone—————————→

Tendon————————→

Muscle—————————→

Nerves

Nerves are the communication pathways of your body. Essentially, nerves work by transmitting electrical impulses between your brain and the rest of your body. There are three types of nerves.

The first type of nerves is called the sensory nerves. Sensory nerves input

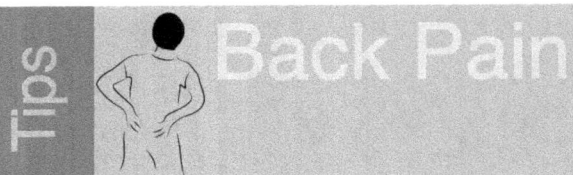

or transfer information (ie: hot/cold, wet/dry, etc...) to the Central Nervous System and brain.

The second type of nerves is called the motor nerves. Motor nerves output or transfer information from the Central Nervous System to the body's muscles or glands (ie: muscle contraction, hormone release, etc...).

The third type of nerve is called an association nerve. Association nerves transfer signals within the Central Nervous System.

The nerves travel from the brain to all parts of the body. As they exit the brain they enter into, and travel through, the spinal column.

The spine is designed to protect the nerves as they travel down the spinal

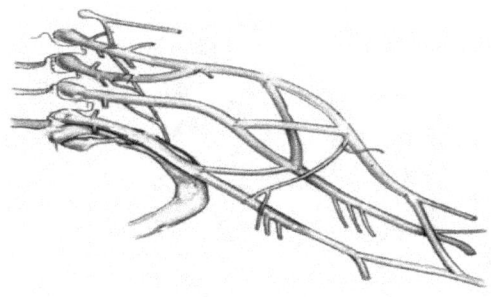

cord before they exit to complete the journey to their destination. As they branch off from the spinal cord, they exit the spine through a canal called the intervertebral foramen.

Treatment

First Things First

If you are having back pain, stop the activity you are doing that is causing your back pain.

This could be as simple as standing up while at work or sitting down while gardening.

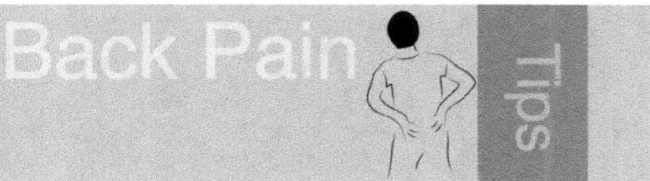

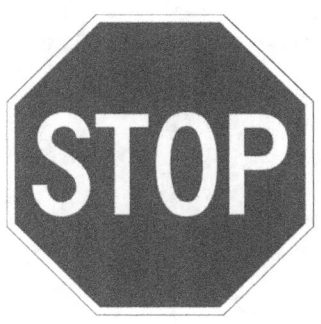

Rest

There used to be an adage that stated that if you hurt your back you should stay in bed for 2 weeks. It was proven that this is the worst thing to do.

The best thing to do is to rest for a short period of time, a few hours to no more than 2 days. Then stop resting and start moving again.

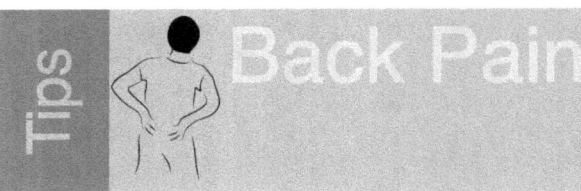

Regaining movement will help you recover faster as well as prevent you from losing muscle strength and endurance.

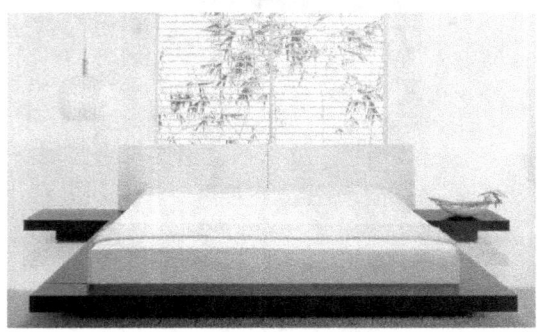

Proper Posture

Sitting, standing and even lying in bed properly can work wonders.

Sit and stand with good posture. This may be painful at first but it will reduce the strain on the injured area.

Back Pain Tips

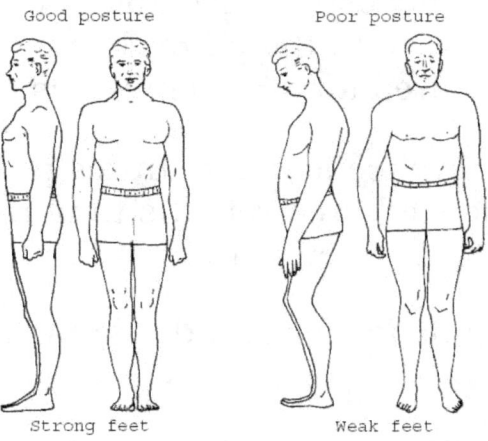

Good posture   Poor posture

Strong feet   Weak feet

Ice

There are two rules to follow when using ice.

1: Use ice first before using heat.

2: Continue using ice for as long as you still feel pain.

To prevent frostbite, place a thin wet

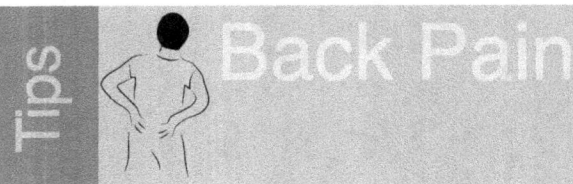

cloth between the ice and your skin. Apply ice to the painful or injured area for 15-20 minutes.

Remove ice for 30 minutes or until the iced area returns to normal temperature.

Reapply ice for an additional 15-20 minutes.

When in doubt use ICE!!!

Heat

There are many times when heat is beneficial to back pain. The best time to use heat is several days or even weeks after an injury. Using heat too soon can make your pain worse.

This is because heat brings more blood and other fluid based nutrients into an area. More blood and fluids in

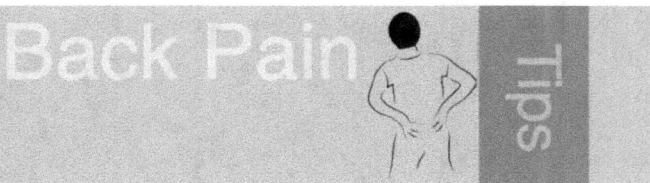

an area means more inflammation. More inflammation usually means more pain.

If you are having more stiffness than pain, then heat is a great choice.

Apply warm heat for 15-20 minutes.

Protect your skin from BURNS!

Ice & Heat Together

Often the best option after the first few days following an injury is a combination of ice and heat. The reason for this is because ice reduces inflammation and pain, and heat increases blood flow and joint motion.

Start with 20 minutes of ice followed

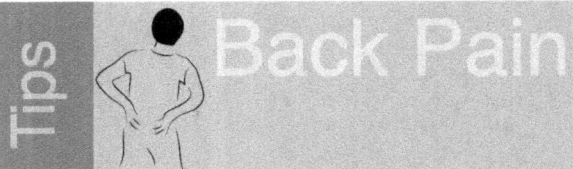

by 30 minutes of nothing to allow your body to return back to normal temperature. Next apply heat for 20 minutes.

You can repeat this cycle several times. Just be sure to allow 30 minutes between the ice and heat to allow your body to naturally return to your normal body temperature.

Drugs

Drugs like Tylenol®, Advil®, Aspirin, etc. mask pain symptoms. They do nothing to eliminate the cause of the pain. They are all intended to reduce inflammation without the use of steroids.

There are potential major side effects that come with using these including

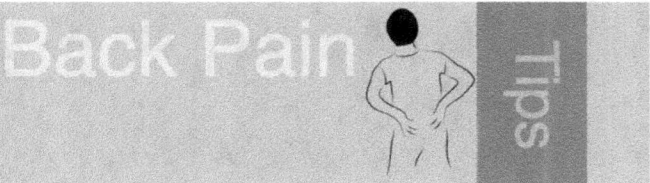

but not limited to:

Gastric bleeding

Cirrhosis of the Liver (long term use)

Death

Never use a higher dose than indicated on the bottle unless directed by your physician.

Massage

Massage therapy, whether performed by a trained massage therapist or a loved one, can be very beneficial to reducing muscle spasms and pain.

There are many types of massage and oftentimes the most effective is deep tissue (myofascial release) or trigger point release techniques.

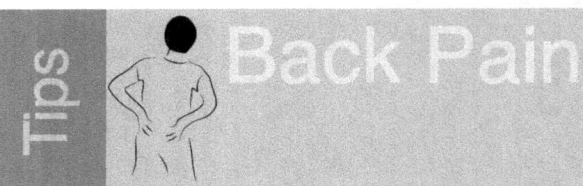

These techniques get deep into the muscles and can cause a muscle spasm to relax and release.

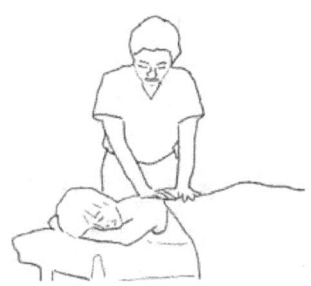

Chiropractic

Chiropractic adjustments are proven to be both highly effective and safe for treating back pain.

When joints in the spine become injured or stop moving properly they produce pain.

Chiropractors adjust the spinal joints

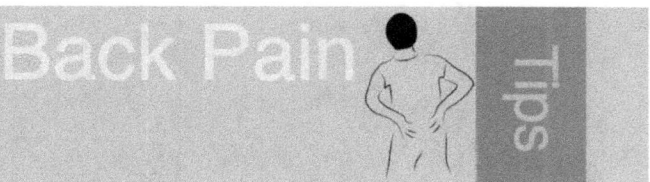

to restore normal joint motion and eliminate pain.

Chiropractors also use other techniques to reduce pain and inflammation.

Chiropractors are the spine experts!

Spinal Decompression

Spinal decompression is a treatment option that can be very beneficial for those with back pain.

There are many forms of spinal decompression from inversion tables (not usually recommended), to computerized mechanical traction tables to Cox® Flexion/Distraction

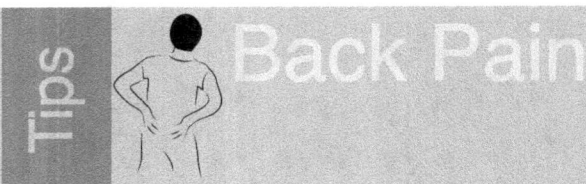

Decompression Technique.

The only spinal decompression technique that both decompresses your spine and restores your range of motion at the same time is the Cox® Flexion/Distraction Decompression Technique.

Check with your chiropractor or neurosurgeon to determine if these techniques will work for you.

Acupuncture

Acupuncture started in Asia 1,000s of years ago. It works by balancing a person's Qi (pronounced chee) or the body's vital energy lines.

Modern medical science does not understand how or why this works but Acupuncture has been proven to be a valid and reliable treatment

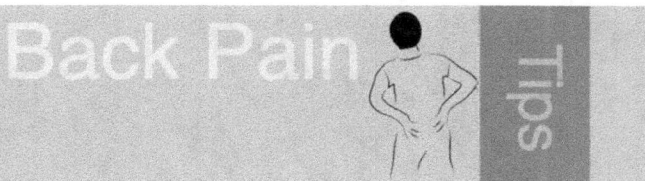

option for managing back pain.

It will not fix the root cause of your symptoms, but it will make the pain more bearable without the use of drugs until the cause of your symptoms has been fixed.

Multi-wavelength lasers can be used to stimulate the body's energy lines instead of needles for those who do not like needles.

Physical Therapy

Physical therapy consists of two different modalities:

- Physiotherapy modalities to block the body's ability to perceive the pain signal temporarily

- Therapeutic exercise to strengthen weak or imbalanced muscles

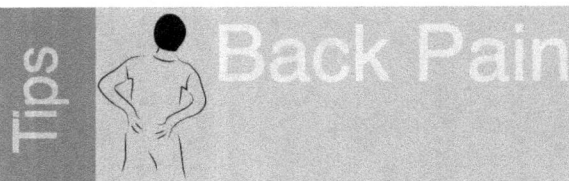

During the first few days after your injury, your Chiropractor will use physiotherapy modalities to bring your pain levels under control without drugs. To achieve maximal results, your Chiropractor will use therapeutic exercise only after your pain and inflammation have been reduced.

Stretches

Stretching can be a very effective means of relaxing a muscle spasm and sometimes even taking pressure off the spine.

All stretching should be performed to your pain level. The stretch should be slightly uncomfortable but not painful. Never bounce.

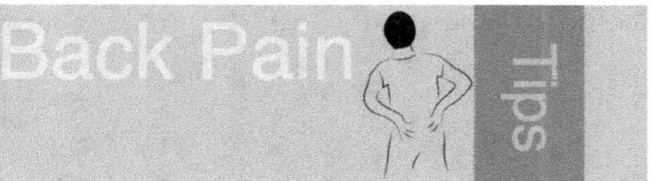

Use a slow and steady pressure. Hold each stretch for 10 to 30 seconds and perform each stretch a minimum of 3 times.

Stretch 2 or 3 times a day.

Everyday!

Knee To Chest Stretch

Lie on your back on the floor or your bed. With both legs straight, slowly bring one leg up to your chest, keeping the other leg as flat on the floor as possible. Use your hands and gently pull your knee closer to your chest.

You can also pull both knees to your

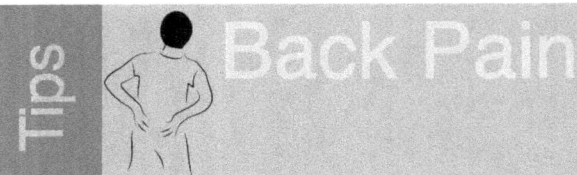

chest at the same time.

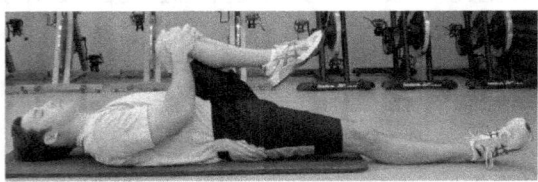

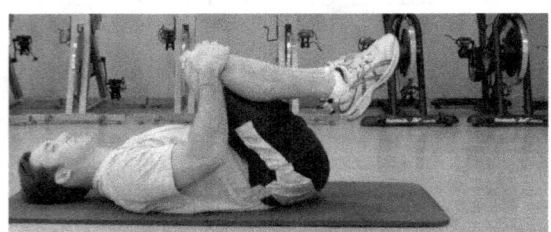

Hamstring Stretch

Sit flat on the floor with your legs straight in front of you. Gently reach down and try to touch your toes.

Grabbing your knees and pulling yourself forward and down may help.

Don't bounce.

Back Pain Tips

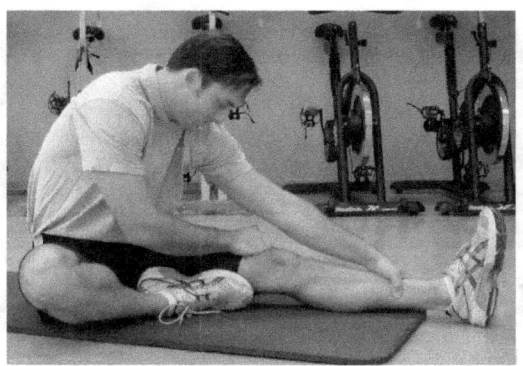

Alternate Hamstring Stretch Using a Chair

An alternative to lying on the floor is to sit on the edge of a chair with one leg straight out in front of you. Slowly reach down your leg toward your ankle. Repeat this stretch for your other leg. Don't bounce.

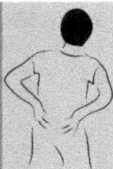 Tips Back Pain

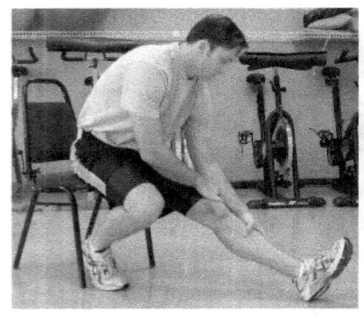 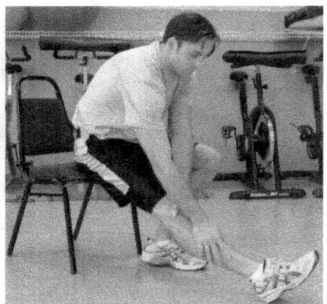

Side To Side

Lay flat on your back on the floor or your bed. Place your feet flat on the floor so your knees are bent. Gently rotate your hips from side to side. Touch your knees to the ground.

Do not use your hands to force your knees to touch the ground if they do not do so easily.

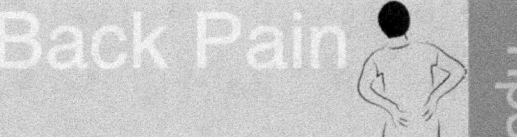

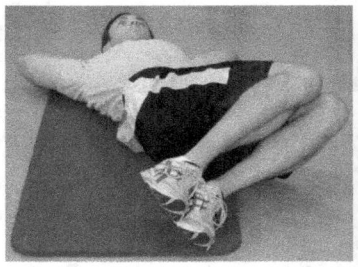 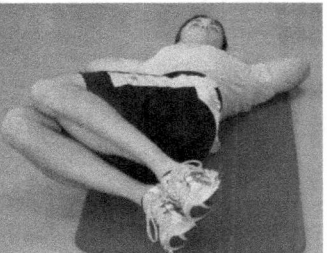

Piriformis Stretch

Lie flat on your back on the floor with one leg bent and the other foot flat on the floor. Cross the bent leg over the knee (rest your foot on your thigh). Next take the back of the leg that is still flat on the floor and gently pull it to your chest.

See the picture below for clarification.

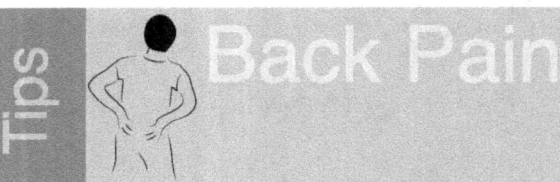

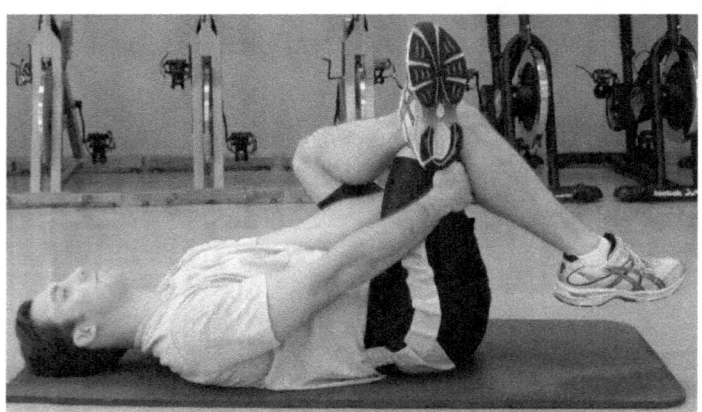

Prevention

An Ounce Of Prevention

The key to preventing back pain is a solid and strong core. The core I am talking about is your mid-section or gut (what we sometimes think of as the stomach).

There are many ways to accomplish

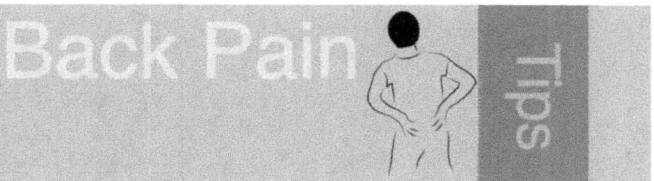

this and we will go over a few of them here.

Waist Circumference

This is a crucial area of your body and not just for back pain. Study after study has shown that the larger your waist size is, the more health problems you will have.

From heart disease, cancer, diabetes, Chron's Disease, liver diseases, kidney dysfunction, sexual

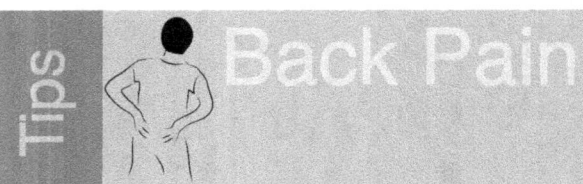

dysfunction, sleeping problems, breathing difficulties, stroke, and yes, even back pain.

Risk factors increase when the waist circumference (pant size) goes up. A woman's waist should be no larger than 35 inches. A man's waist should be no larger than 40 inches.

These sizes are not goals you should target. They are statistical numbers that were derived from hundreds of studies and they show where the highest risk occurs for acquiring one or more disease or health problem for the largest number of Americans.

What needs to be remembered is that waist size is only one risk factor affecting your health and there are many more risk factors that you should be aware. That's why even women with a 32 inch waist and men

Back Pain Tips

with a 37 inch waist are still at a high incidence of these health conditions.

The real dilemma is that over 50% of all Americans are overweight or obese and are ticking time bombs. It also means there are more people at risk for all of these health conditions than there are those who are not at risk.

For these reasons alone, maintaining a healthy waist circumference of less than 32 inches for women and 36 inches for men is important, but there is also another consideration to keep in mind...

Having a slim waist will make you look good and feel good!

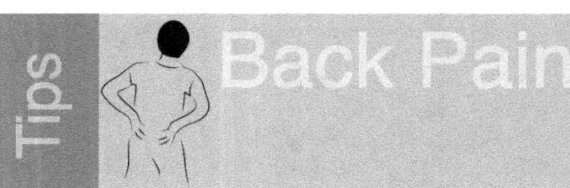

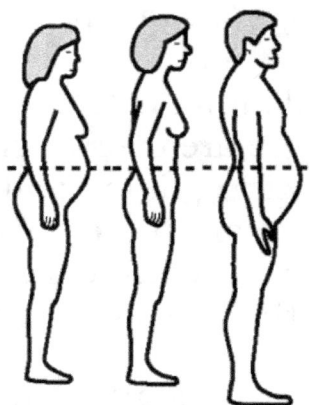

Proper Nutrition

Proper diet is crucial in preventing back pain. Many foods, such as breads and pastas, are known to increase inflammation and pain levels and to keep them elevated longer.

Also, the large amount of man-made chemicals consumed every day in the processed foods that the average

American consumer eats in such large quantities causes increased risk for both back pain and health problems in general.

Good Foods

There are foods that can actually help lower inflammation while also helping maintain healthy blood sugar levels.

Eating foods that improve your health and vitality rather than foods that don't reduces your risk of acquiring back pain and other health conditions and as an added benefit, it

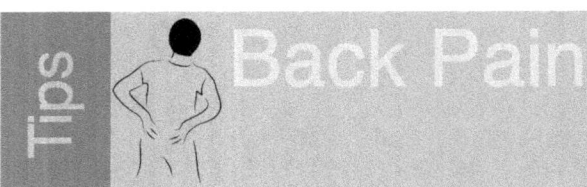

will also help increase your longevity.

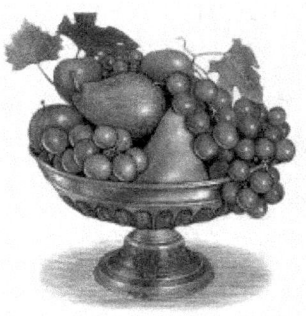

Nuts And Seeds
(preferably raw)

Almonds / Pecans / Walnuts

Macadamia / Brazil / Pine Nuts

Hempseeds

Pumpkin Seeds

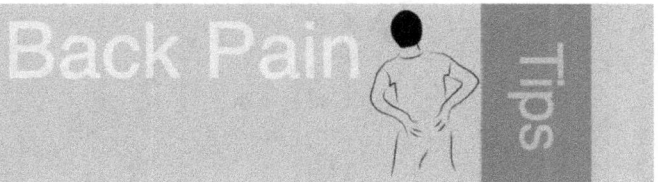

Chia Seeds

Flaxseeds

Beans (black, kidney, lima)

Fruits (organic is best)

Blueberries

Raspberries

Blackberries

Strawberries

Acai / Goji Berries

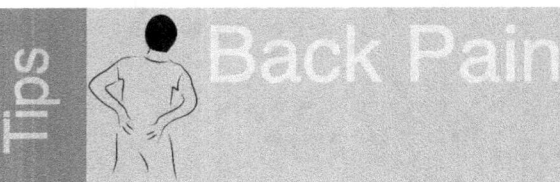

Lemon

Lime

Apples

Cherries

Pears

Kiwi

Fruits With Simple Moderation

Oranges

Mangos

Melons

Pineapple

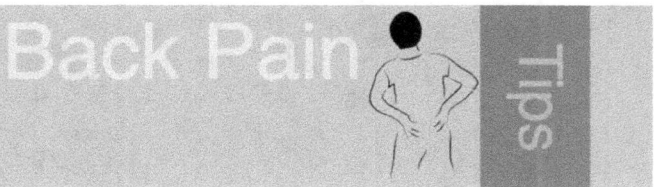

Bananas

Papaya

Meat (wild game or grass fed)

Beef

Deer

Bison

Chicken

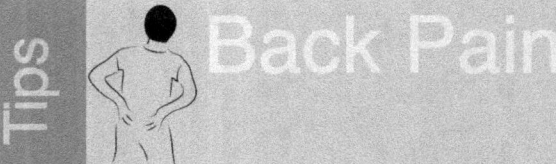

Turkey

Fresh Wild Fish

Wild Game

Lamb

Cage Free Eggs

Vegetables

All green leafy vegetables

Eggplant

Zucchini

Radishes

Celery

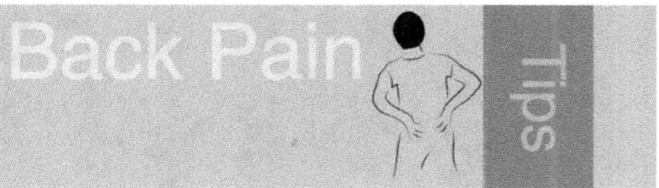

Kale

Green Beans

Bell peppers

Cucumber

Onions

Mushrooms

Asparagus

Broccoli

Brussels Sprouts

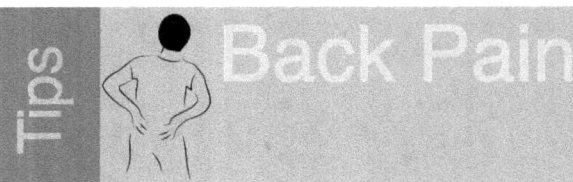

Condiments

Sea Salt

Apple Cider Vinegar

Salsa

Guacamole

Balsamic Vinegar

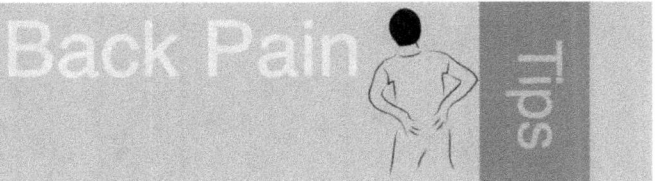

Mustard

All Herbs and Spices

Organic flavorings

Foods To Avoid

These foods can increase your pain.

Breads

Pastas

Rice

Dairy

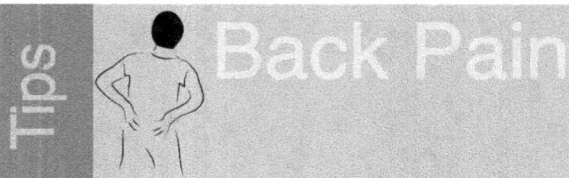

Cheese

Peanuts

Fast Food

Deep Fried Foods

Pork

Soft drinks

Beverages

Water (purified and free from chlorine and fluoride)

Herbal Teas

Raw Vegetable Juices (Juice-o-Matic)

Fresh squeezed fruit juice (limit this due to high sugar content)

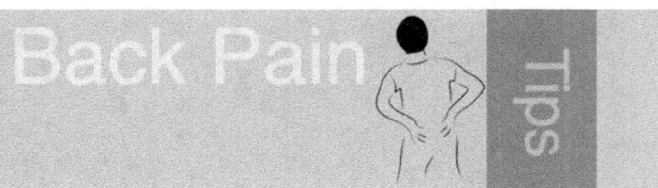

Fermented Beverages (red wines and darker beers) in moderation

How Much Water?

This is a common question with a relatively easy answer.

A sedentary adult male who weighs 200 pounds should consume between 48 and 62 ounces of water (about 6 to 8 classes) a day. This is pure water, not sugary juices or sodas.

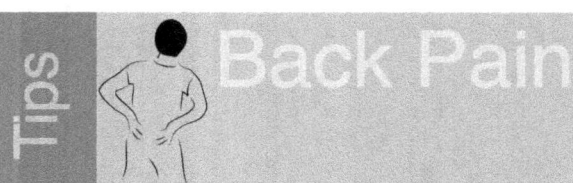

Sugar spikes insulin levels causing fat to be stored and caffeine acts as a diuretic causing you to lose water and become dehydrated.

For a 200 pound male who exercises or works in a hot environment, or sweats a lot, more water is required.

The general rule is 1 liter of water (about 33 ounces) per hour is needed to maintain hydration lost from sweating for those who are in high heat areas or are performing strenuous activities.

Females need slightly less water per day unless they are performing strenuous activities or are exposed to high temperatures. Then about 1 liter (about 33 ounces) per hour is appropriate to replace fluids lost to sweat.

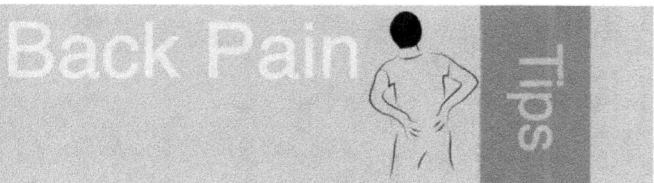

A good rule to follow is, if you are sweating due to either intense activity or heat and are thirsty, you are already dehydrated. Drink continuously during these times.

Stretching

In addition to being part of the treatment for back pain, stretching is also a preventative measure.

You should continue to perform the following stretches everyday to prevent back pain in the future.

Knee to Chest

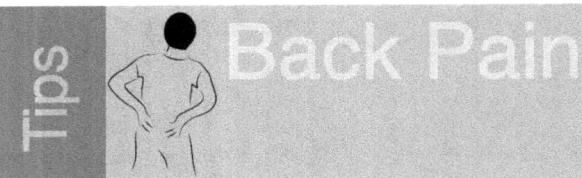

Hamstring Stretch

Alternative Hamstring Stretch

Side to Side

Piriformis Stretch

Exercise

You need 30 minutes of strenuous physical activity in the form of structured exercise every day to maintain a healthy body weight and a high level of overall health.

Since we are focused on low back pain and the prevention of low back pain, the following exercises were

Back Pain Tips

designed specifically to strengthen the core muscles. They are simple, effective, and efficient.

Disclaimer: Always consult your doctor before beginning any exercise program. Even a program as simple as this.

Walking

Walking is a good starting exercise for people who live a sedentary life.

Walking is an effective exercise for preventing many health conditions and especially back pain.

Walking can help you lose your gut and help you strengthen your core.

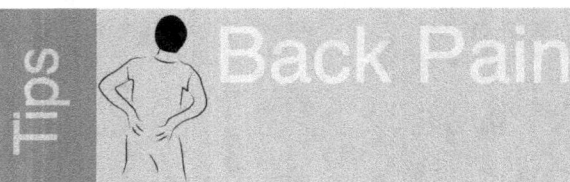

In order for walking to be effective as an exercise, it must be performed at a brisk pace, 3 miles per hour, and must be performed for at least 30 minutes per day.

One of the best forms of walking is called Heavy Hands® and was developed by Leonard Swartz, MD in the early 1980s.

Heavy Hands® books and equipment are available at most retailers and on the internet. For about $40 you get the book and the basic equipment.

It's best to walk outside as much as possible as you get Vitamin D from sunshine and the fresh air can be invigorating.

If you are using the Heavy Hands® routine and must walk indoors, you

Back Pain Tips

do not need a treadmill. You can walk in place and get as much or more exercise as you would on the most expensive treadmill.

Another good walking program is called 10,000 Steps® which was developed in 2001 by David Satcher, MD and C. Everett Coop, MD.

Suck It In

Ab-Brace-Hollow is an exercise in both proper breathing (belly breathing) and core strength.

Lie on your back with your feet on the floor and your knees in the air.

Next force your low back down into the floor. This is called a posterior

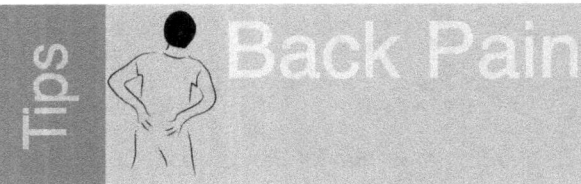

pelvic tilt.

Now squeeze the sides of your stomach together. If you are having difficulty getting these muscles to do anything, poke them with your finger. This will send a signal from the nerve to the brain (remember that connection) telling your brain to contract that muscle.

Now suck your belly button down. Try to suck it in so far back that it touches your spine.

And lastly breathe. Force your stomach up when you take a breath in. Do this while holding the previous steps firm.

Don't worry if this seems difficult at first. For most people this exercise will take some practice to perfect.

Back Pain 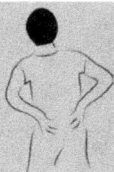 Tips

Do this 3 or 4 times a day. Practice this until you are walking around with your core tight all the time.

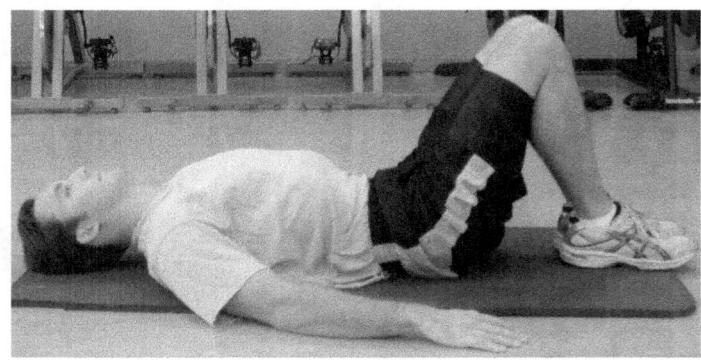

Dead Bug

This exercise is designed to both strengthen the abdominal muscles and to increase their endurance.

Start by lying flat on your back with your arms and legs straight up in the air. This makes you look like a "dead bug".

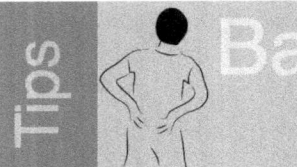

Lower your left leg towards the floor, do not let your leg touch the floor. At the same time, lower your right arm to the floor, again without touching the floor. Pause for one second and bring your leg and arm back to the starting position.

Next, lower you right leg and your left arm, pause and then return to the starting position.

Perform 15 repetitions for both left and right combinations.

Perform 3 sets of 15 repetitions every day.

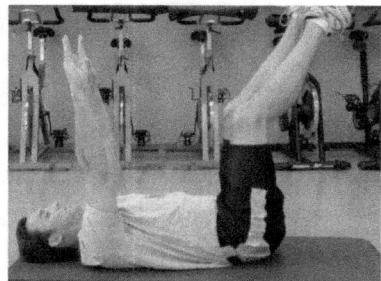

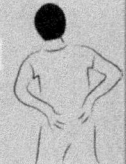
Back Pain
Tips

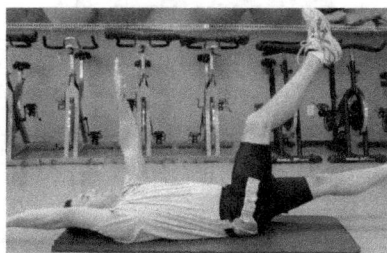

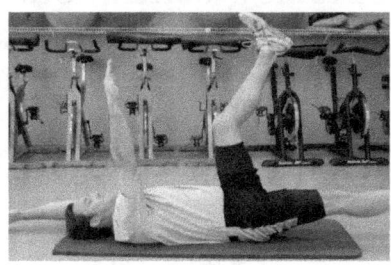

Cat And Camel

This is a combination stretch and strengthening exercise. It helps to increase motion in your spinal joints

Position yourself on all fours as if you were going to crawl around. Use the Ab-Brace-Hollow technique you learned earlier and tighten your abdominal muscles.

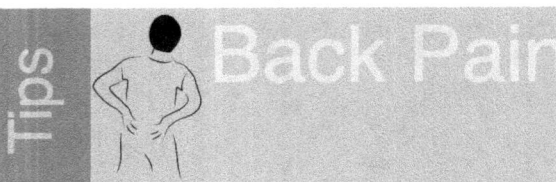

Arch your back up into the air (like a cat) and tuck your chin into your chest. Hold for 3 seconds. Next drop your belly to the floor and look up to the sky. Hold for 3 seconds.

Do this in a slow continuous motion. Don't pause for more than 3 seconds in any one position and do not bend your arms.

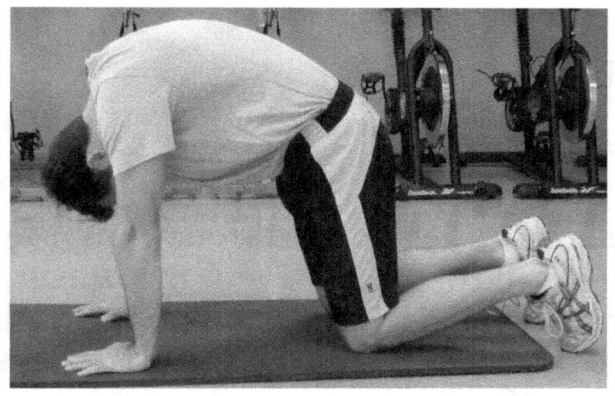

Back Pain 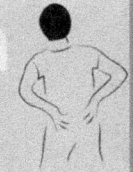 Tips

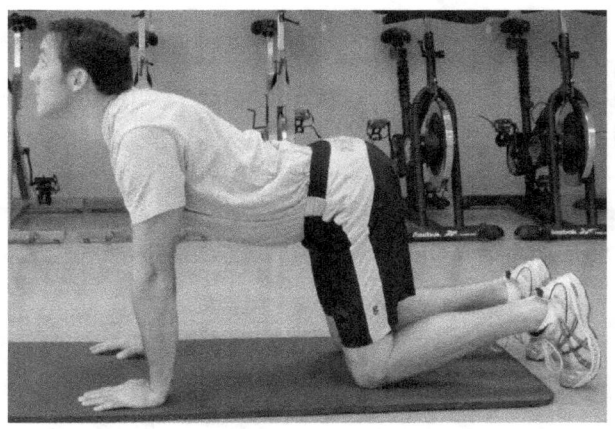

Be Super

This exercise is great exercise for the muscles that run along your spine.

Start by lying on your chest with your arms and legs outstretched, just like Superman. Keep your arms and legs straight, raise your left leg and right arm off the floor at the same time. Pause for 3 seconds. Lower your arm

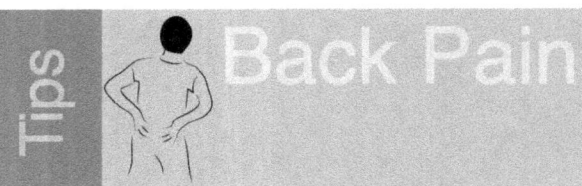

and leg to the floor.

Next, raise your right leg and left arm off the floor at the same time. Pause for 3 seconds. Lower your arm and leg to the floor.

Perform 15 repetitions for each arm and leg combination.

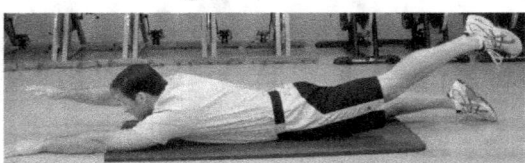

Build A Strong Bridge

Bridging exercises are very effective at increasing spinal strength.

Lie with your back and feet flat on the floor. Bend your knees.

Raise your pelvis off the floor while keeping your feet flat. From your knee to your shoulder should make a

Back Pain Tips

straight line. Hold the position for a count of one. Your hamstring muscles should not be contracted.

Perform 15 repetitions.

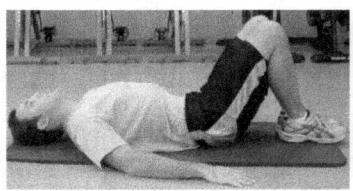 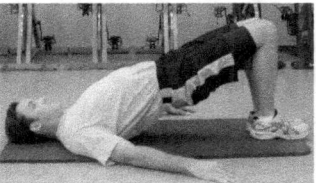

It's Good To Crawl Around

One of the first and most important exercises we do after we are born is crawling. Although babies don't consider it exercise.

Start on all fours as if you were going to crawl around on the ground.

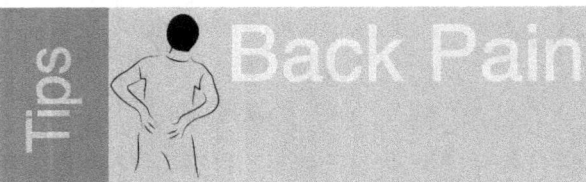

Tighten your abdominal muscles using Ab-Brace-Hollow.

Extend your left leg behind you and your right arm in front of you. Your body should make a straight line from your shoulders to your toes. Pause for 3 seconds and then bring your arm and leg back to the floor.

Extend your left leg behind you and your right arm in front of you. Pause for 3 seconds and then bring your arm and leg back to the floor.

Perform 15 repetitions on each arm and leg.

Back Pain 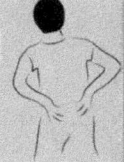 Tips

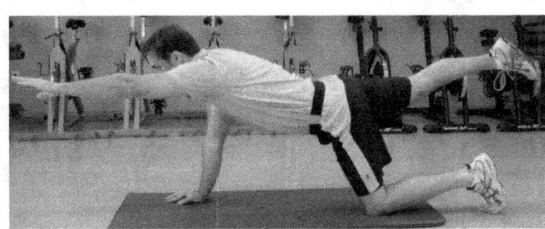

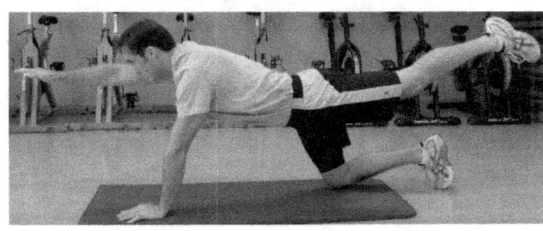

Just Keep Swimming

Swimming and other water exercises
are good forms of exercise that
almost anyone can perform. They are
low to no impact exercises.

Water is an excellent medium to
exercise in because your body is
more than 55% water. It will weigh
less and gain support while

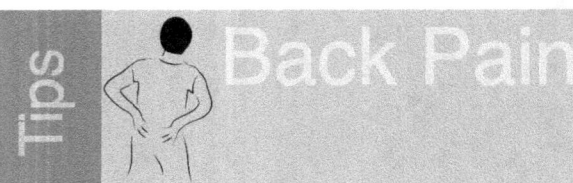

immersed. However, even though
your body weighs less, the exertion
will be the same or more because of
the drag of the water on the body.

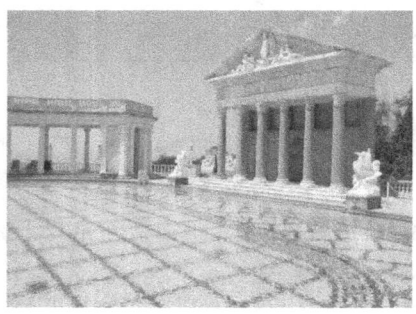

Proper Mattress

Sleep is crucial for a healthy life as it is the time that the body repairs and rebuilds itself. A mattress that is too old, too hard, too soft or too anything else that causes you to lose sleep or awaken in pain, needs to be replaced.

A mattress should be chosen for its comfort and spine support. The

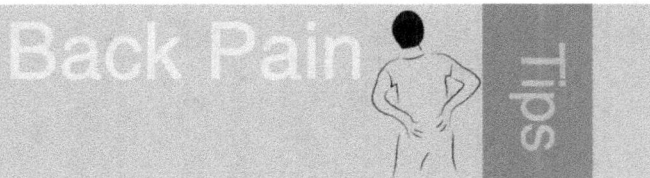

quality of your sleep experience is more important than the look, brand name or top covering.

Consider one of the memory foam mattresses, or an adjustable sleep number mattress, a water bed or even an adjustable bed.

Purchase the best mattress that you can afford.

Pillows

Pillow selection is as important as mattress selection is for sleep quality. Pillows are designed to provide both support and cushioning.

Back sleepers should use a medium support pillow to support the curvature of their upper spine and provide support under their head,

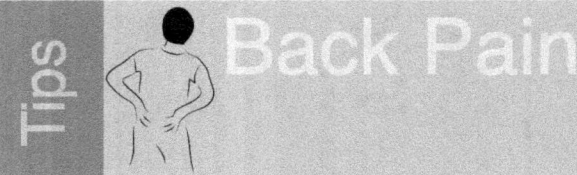

neck and shoulders.

Side sleepers should use a pillow that contours and cradles their neck and provides an even sleeping surface. Side sleeper pillows need to keep the body in a horizontal line.

Stomach sleepers should use a soft pillow so that their head and neck aren't turned unnaturally to either side.

Proper Sleeping Position

You should sleep in a position that is comfortable to you but also one that will help reduce back pain.

The ideal position is sleeping flat on your back. This position reduces the amount of stress and strain on your

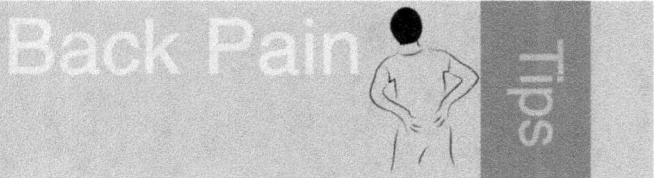

neck and back.

The second best sleep position is on your side. Sleep on a pillow that supports your neck and put a pillow behind you to add spine support.

If at all possible, avoid sleeping on your stomach.

Supplements

There is an enormous body of information, and controversy, on the subject of supplementing your diet with vitamins, minerals and other food supplements.

Consider this: Why do farmers add supplements to their soil, ranchers give supplements to their livestock,

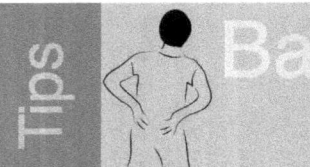

and food manufacturers add supplements to their products?

They add vitamin and mineral supplements because the soil is barren and lacks key nutritional ingredients. This means that since the entire food chain starts in the soil, everything in the food chain is lacking in vitamins and minerals and must be supplemented at each stage.

Proper supplementation is too large and complex a subject to go into great detail here, however, there are vitamin and mineral supplements that are beneficial to both treating and preventing back pain.

Omega-3 fish oils are anti-inflammatory supplements.

Vitamin B complex is good for increasing energy levels and proper

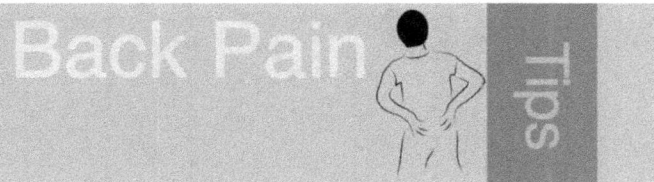

cellular function.

Vitamin D is an integral component of bone health as well as a good anti-inflammatory.

"Foot" Essentials

There is a causal link between the care of your feet and the amount of pain you experience in your back, knees and hips.

Proper footwear is crucial for reducing and eliminating back pain.

Footwear comes in all shapes and

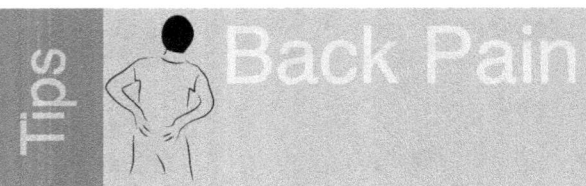

designs. Most have a purpose and are intended for a specific use but there are some that are strictly for style and are wardrobe specific.

Choosing Proper Footwear

Footwear should be chosen for the specific activity that you will be participating in.

Manufacturer's design each style of shoe and each style of sneaker for specific activities. It is self destructive

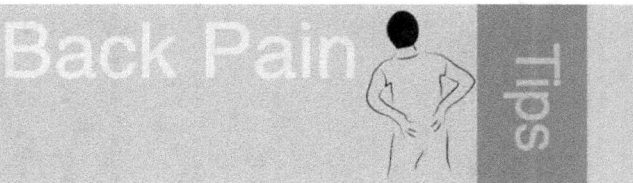

to wear dress shoes or high heels to run in a marathon. Although not destructive, it's not exactly stylish to wear running shoes while wearing a tuxedo or evening dress.

Running shoes are designed with extra shock absorbing capability and should be used for running.

Walking shoes are designed with their shock absorbing material distributed specifically to the way in which the foot strikes when walking.

Basketball shoes are designed with tread material, tread pattern, shock absorption and ankle support designed for the game of basketball.

Tennis shoes are designed for a specific type of play surface (dirt,

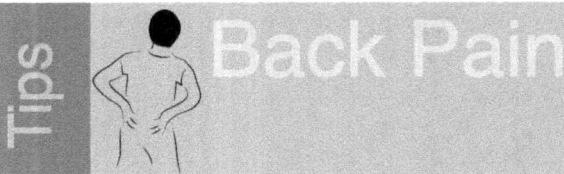

clay, grass, etc...)

Golf shoes are designed for use on a golf course (or to aerate your lawn).

Cross-training shoes are designed for all around activities.

Shoes designed for skateboards can also be used as walking shoes because they have good arch support and are flat on the bottom.

Proper Fitting

The task of properly sizing and fitting footwear can be arduous due to the multitude of shoe manufacturers, styles and costs.

There are a lot of things to consider when fitting shoes. Functionally, there is length, width, arch support, ankle support, heel and toe fit, angle

Back Pain Tips

of the shoe, material and purpose that must be considered.

Aesthetically, there is style, color, tread pattern, logo (branding), etc...

The easiest way to find and fit proper footwear is to go a specialty shoe store. The clerks are usually trained in proper sizing and fitting of the different footwear and can help you make the correct decision (or not).

When To Replace Your Old Shoes

Knowing when to replace your footwear is tricky question. Footwear gets comfortable and are like old friends. You don't want to toss them out too soon and not get your money's worth but you don't want to wait too long and develop back pain.

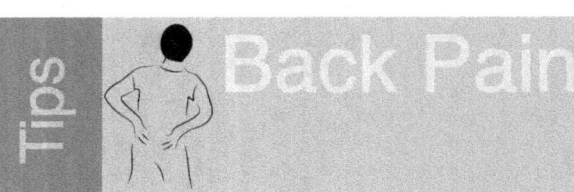

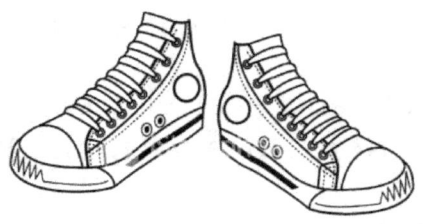

Shoe Rules:

If they have holes, toss them.

If there's no tread left, toss them.

If they lean to one side, toss them.

If they hurt to wear, toss them.

If your toes are starting to curl because you're growing, toss them.

If you develop knee pain and don't know why, try new footwear.

When in doubt REPLACE them.

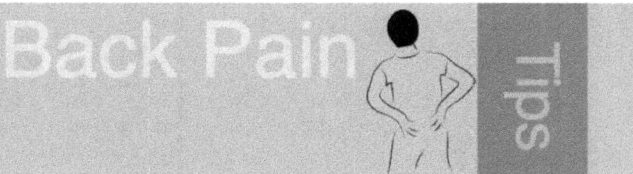

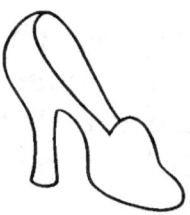 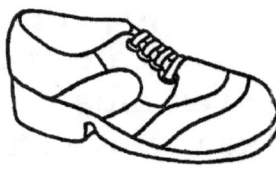

Gardening

A lot of people enjoy gardening and other activities where they repetitively hunch over, kneel down or crouch on their ankles.

All three of these positions are uncomfortable and can lead to muscle cramps and spasms. Worse, they can lead to a sprain or a strain

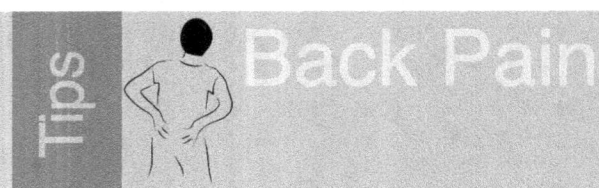

even after a short period of time.

It is best to perform these activities from a seated position. In cases where you must be near ground level, make use of a step stool or even a plastic milk case.

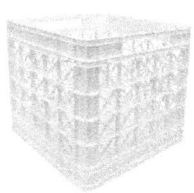

Sitting On The Job

A lot of people are required to sit for long periods of time as a function of their jobs.

Examples include truck drivers, pilots, office workers, etc...

Sitting for long periods of time compresses the discs of the spine

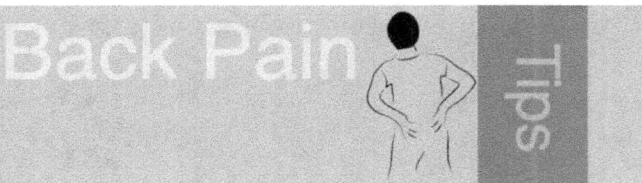

while also allowing the muscles of the spine to atrophy. In addition, the discs of the spine require movement for the nutrients to reach them.

If your work requires long periods of sitting, every hour you should stand up, slowly perform 5 deep knee bends, 5 overhead arm lifts and then follow these with a brief walk.

Sitting Position

When sitting in a chair it is very important to use proper sitting posture to help prevent back pain.

The best sitting position for your spine is with your buttock right at the edge of the seat, shoulders back, chest out slightly, head held high and the palms of your hands rotated so

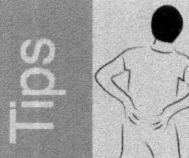 Back Pain

Tips

that they are facing forward and even slightly out to the side.

Use extreme caution if your chair has wheels or the floor is slippery.

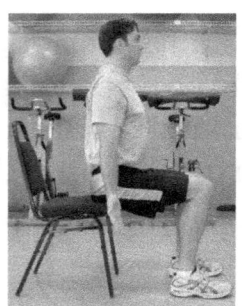 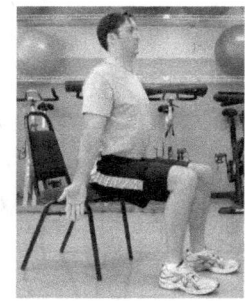

Conclusion

The best chance of reducing back pain is prevention of back pain. If you follow the instructions in this book you will reduce your frequency, duration and intensity of back pain throughout your life.

The main keys are proper exercise, proper posture, proper weight

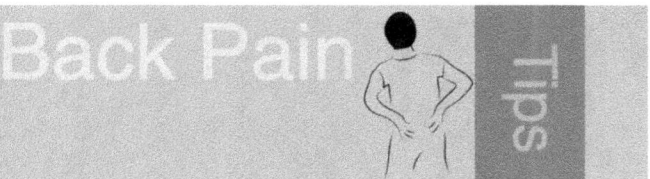

management, proper nutrition, and chiropractic preventative treatments.

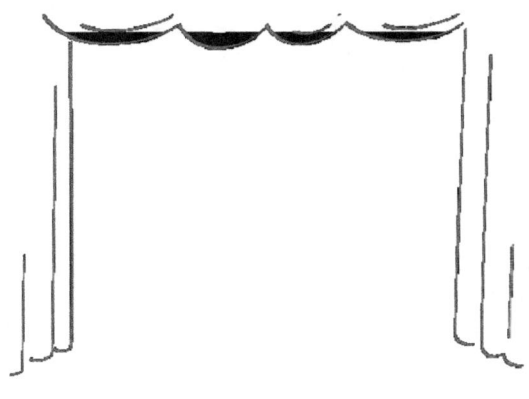

Notes:

Notes:

Follow Along With Dr. Walsh

To stay abreast of the latest updates in the chiropractic, acupuncture and medical fields visit:

Dr. Walsh's website:

www.newsmyrnaspine.com

Dr. Walsh's health blog:

www.docwalsh.com

To learn the latest in accident and injury treatment and prevention:

www.thewhiplashchronicles.com

If you have been in an accident and don't know what to do first:

www.mywhiplashreport.com

www.ingramcontent.com/pod-product-compliance
Lightning Source LLC
Chambersburg PA
CBHW072213280526
45788CB00002B/1001